21 Myths about Drugs and Medicines

Merlvin Moyo

DEDICATION

To all the patients, friends and family members that ask me these sorts of
questions every day

Contents

Foreword

Let's start off with a disclaimer: I am a pharmacist. I work with patients and drugs every day. I earn a living from dealing in drugs and medicines. For some people that is a problem. They assume that since I have a vested interest in the use of drugs by patients then I cannot be relied upon to give an objective, reliable account of anything related to drugs. I accept that some people will have this view.

On the other hand, if for some reason you wanted to find out about a particular religion or culture we have to assume that you would not just rely on the criticisms of those without any experience of it. It is likely that you would spend at least some time getting the views of those with experience of that culture.

As a pharmacist I might not have tried drugs myself, but the training that pharmacists get both at university and post-qualification gives them a deeper understanding of drugs than you can usually get from a few days' search on the internet. You owe it to yourself to hear what your pharmacist has to say about them.

The healing properties of medicines have granted them a mystique since the earliest days of recorded human history. In primitive societies the lack of a sound scientific basis for understanding the mechanisms of action of the active components led many people to ascribe spiritual properties to various natural products, both organic and inorganic. Even in relatively developed societies, one only has to look at the pharmacopoeias from a few decades ago to appreciate the level of ignorance about medicines that existed until recently.

It would be easy to argue that this ignorance is a mark of times past.

However, any medical professional will have come across statements from patients that show that there remains a great need for educating ordinary men and women about the millions of tablets, capsules and liquids that they take into their bodies on a daily basis.

This book represents some of the myths I have come across in my practice. They are not listed in any order of priority.

As a disclaimer I have to add that while every care has been taken to ensure that the information provided is accurate, the understanding of that information might at any time be superseded by new research or better interpretation of existing data. The author cannot be held responsible for such changes. In addition to this, as the book is intended for general information for non-health personnel, the author has chosen to make use of a variety of sources in the public domain, including non-professional resources, where these are deemed fairly accurate for the purpose of the discussions in the myth under consideration. This is purely for convenience as it enables the reader, if interested, to look up further any information discussed in the book. Health professionals and students are advised to refer to standard peer-reviewed publications if they wish to check information for accuracy and use in patient care.

A final point is that although I am a pharmacist by profession, the opinions I express in this book are not to be taken as a substitute for a proper consultation with your qualified pharmacist or doctor if you have need for specific advice about a personal problem or one relating to someone you know. Always consult a health professional before taking any medication for the first time, if in doubt, if there is a need to continue medication for extended periods or if there is a worsening of symptoms.

1: "All Drugs are Bad; but Medicines are All Good"

"Hi. I'd like to have a word with the chemist, please," a customer says to a health assistant.

"Sure, I'll get her for you. Can I ask what it's in relation to."

"I just want to ask her about a personal medical problem. I want to check if this medicine (holding up a pack of some popular brand) is okay with my medication."

The assistant goes over to the pharmacist and tells her about the request. The pharmacist comes aver and starts going through some routine questions with the patient.

"Good afternoon. Sarah tells me you want to find out about this medicine. May I ask what you need it for?"

"Certainly. It's for pain relief. I've already tried a number of different things and they are not touching the pain."

"Really? … I need to check a few things first; just to make sure this is suitable for you. What sort of pain do you have?"

"Well; It's over here, and it feels like …," the patient responds, going into some detail to explain how severe it is, how long she's had it for and what she's already tried for it.

"I see. That's useful information," says the pharmacist. "May I ask what other drugs you are taking at the moment?"

"Drugs? I don't take any drugs," is the surprised response from the patient.

"I'm sorry. I meant to ask what medicines you are taking," the pharmacist explains. "We use the terms interchangeably."

"Oh!" responds a visibly relieved patient. She then goes on to provide the requested information.

In practice you would hardly ever get the last question from the pharmacist; as written above. Most pharmacists use the terms "medicines" or "medication' in conversation with patients; yet when they speak amongst themselves they talk almost exclusively about drugs.

Patients generally associate "drugs" with illicit active substances such as crystal meth, crack, heroin, ecstasy and weed; amongst a multitude of others. They do not regard their blood pressure, asthma or diabetes medication as "drugs". However, a simple check in most dictionaries show that the definition of "drug" is much more inclusive.

The Oxford English Dictionary defines a drug (noun) as "a medicine or other substance which has a physiological effect when ingested or otherwise introduced into the body." It offers a secondary definition of a drug as "a substance taken for its narcotic or stimulant effects, often illegally."

The main definition therefore encompasses what people commonly refer to as "medicines" in whatever form they come: tablets, capsules, creams, ointments, liquids, powders, injections, patches, sprays or even implants. With this understanding, substances of abuse are then seen as a subset within the wider definition.

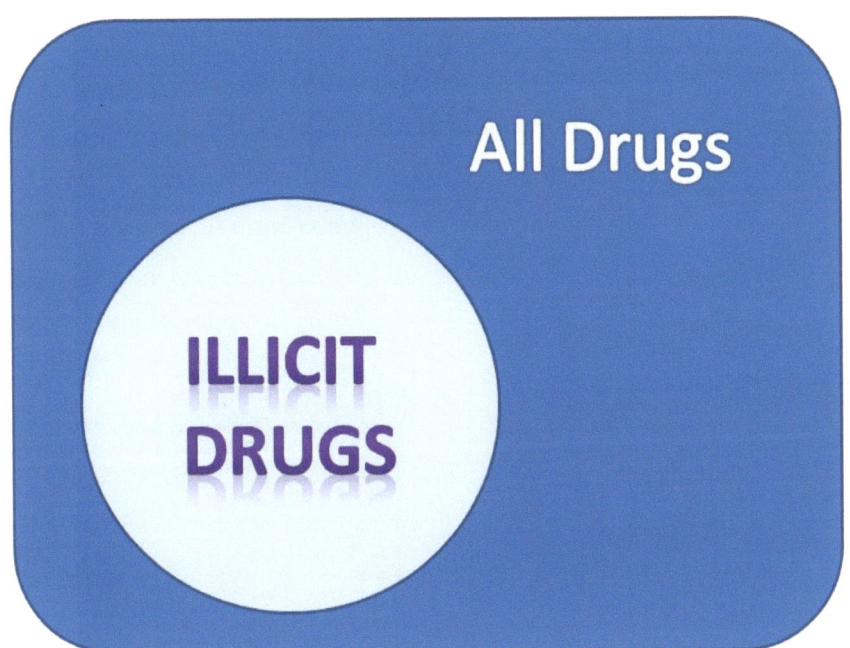

Figure 1 Drugs versus Illicit Drugs

It is important to understand this for several reasons:

1. In regular conversation, when ordinary people talk about "medicines" they generally refer to liquid formulations of drugs:

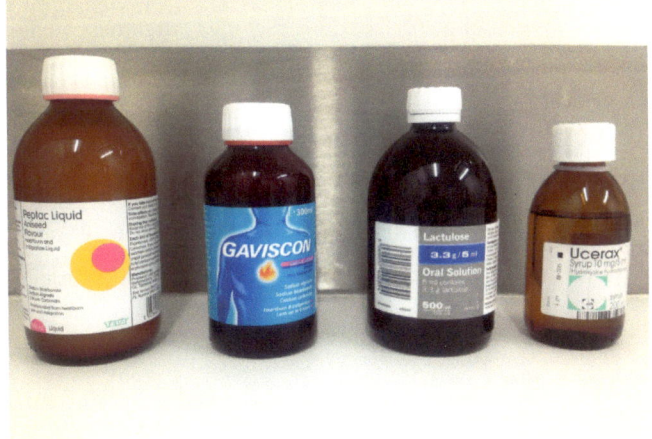

Figure 2 What some people refer to as "medicines"

In reality the dictionary makes clear that a drug can be the same thing as a medicine since it defines a medicine as "a drug or other preparation for the treatment or prevention of disease." (Ibid).

It is important to note that the definition of "medicine" above is centred on the fact that it is the *prepared* form of the drug that is referred to as the medicine, irrespective of the nature of that preparation. Thus, if I have pure Paracetamol powder in the laboratory, it is a drug but is probably not in the best form for administering to a patient. If I take that same powder, add a diluent such as starch powder, put a preservative of some sort, add a disintegrating and lubricating agents, then compress the mixture into tablet form in a press; I have turned the drug into a medicine. Of course it is possible to argue that the original powder was already a medicine since you could package it into sachets for dissolution in a suitable liquid before intake by a patient; but I think you get the picture.

There is another aspect to the definition of a medicine that is evident. The medicine is defined as a "drug **or other preparation**.." Thus drugs are a subset of a wider pool of things referred to as medicines. Non-drug medication includes vaccines (made from parts of viruses or from live attenuated forms) and even, at times, special foods.

2. Some regularly abused drugs actually have genuine uses in medical care; in the form of legal pharmaceutical versions. Take, for example, diamorphine, which is the pharmaceutical name for what is popularly referred to as heroin. Rightly used, it plays an important role in pain relief. On the street, people use it to stimulate their opioid receptors in the brain and to get a feeling of euphoria. Marijuana is a plant that is commonly abused in the form skunk,

weed, cakes and other forms for its euphoria-inducing properties. It might therefore come as a surprise to some people that the cannabinoids that it contains – the reason for its popularity – can be extracted and used in the medical field. There is a licensed formulation of this active component used in a drug for multiple sclerosis.

3. A lot of drug abuse is centred on legal medication. The stereotypical drug addict is not truly representative of the number of people that abuse drugs out there. Not all drug abuse is centred on syringes, needles, pans and flames.

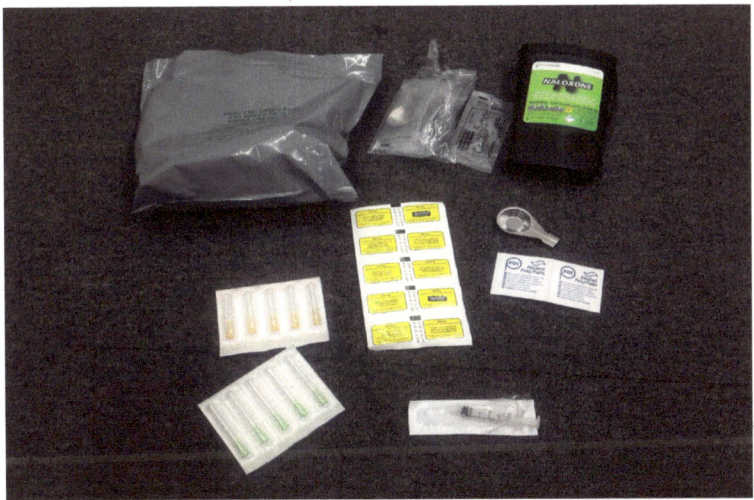

Figure 3 Paraphernalia given as part of a Needle and Syringe Exchange Scheme

Some people go to incredible lengths to get prescription drugs from medical professionals. Opiates (fentanyl, morphone, oxycodone etc) and benzodiazepines (e.g. diazepam) tend to be their drugs of choice. Not only do some feign illness with the prescription of these in mind, others will try to buy or steal them from patients that have genuinely got them on prescription from doctors. In extreme cases it in not uncommon in the medical and retail pharmacy worlds to come across people that steal prescription pads with the intention of writing forged prescriptions for such drugs. It is noteworthy that these drugs are often implicated in the premature deaths of high-profile celebrities.

Of course the abuse does not just occur with prescription drugs. If you regularly buy common dihydrocodeine or codeine-containing painkillers over the counter, it is possible that you might be abusing them. Medicines such as Co-Codamol, Solpadeine®, Nurofen Plus®, Paramol® or Paracodol® are licensed for use only over short periods of time in the UK. In most cases they come with a big warning sign that their use must be limited to short periods.

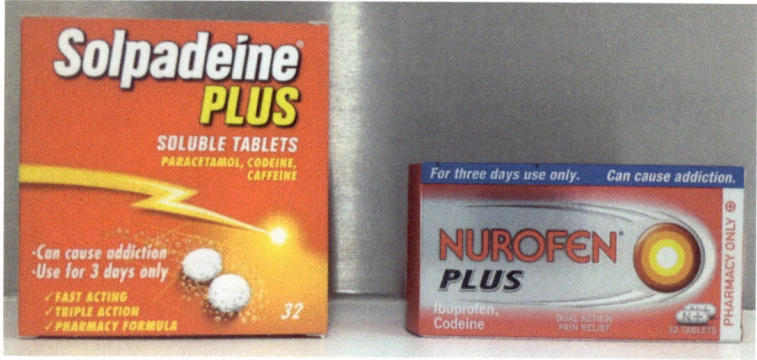

Figure 4 Common codeine-containing medicines with warning signs

One of the responsibilities of pharmacy teams is to spot potential abuse of such drugs and to try to help patients in a professional way.

What are the implications of the above discussion? It should be evident that is not possible to say that all drugs are "bad" and all medicines are "good" in a generic sense. A drug and a medicine can be the same thing. For drugs that have a proven medical use, it is quite often the manner in which they are used that determines the "goodness" or "badness" thereof. If a drug has a genuine medical use but is being used to induce feelings of euphoria, calmness or prevent withdrawal symptoms other than in accordance with a proper prescription from a qualified professional, then it is likely being abused. Drugs, in the right context, are good. Medicines, used inappropriately, are bad.

2: "Herbal Medicines do not have Side Effects"

I am a believer in herbal medicines and other "natural medicines". I firmly believe that the treatment of many ailments that plague human society would not be where it is today if it were not for the discoveries of the wonderful properties of various natural products over the several millennia during which humans have been on this planet. In fact, any first-year pharmacy student should be able to give you some examples of important drugs that are derived from plants.

Among the classic examples are aspirin, derived from the willow tree; and digoxin, which is derived from the foxglove plant. The former has many uses spanning pain relief and prevention of formation of blood clots. New benefits are regularly discovered. At the time of writing this chapter (August 2014), there are rumours of benefits from Aspirin intake in cancer. Digoxin, on the other hand, is used for certain types of irregular heartbeat.

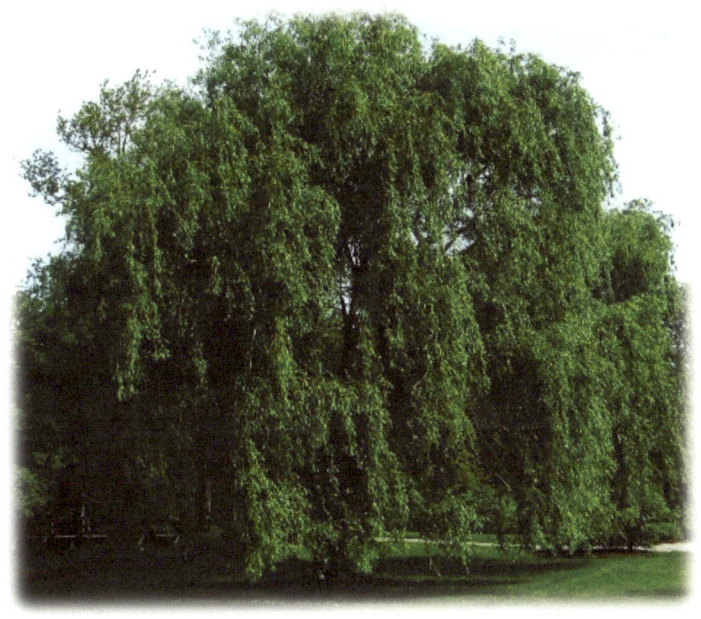

Figure 5 Willow Tree

Now, there's a big difference between saying that I am a believer in herbal medicines, for the reasons stated above, and saying that the use of such medicines is completely without risk; which is what some people believe. The belief is that "natural remedies", unlike "artificial drugs", do not run the risk of producing side effects in the user. A lot of companies play on this ignorance amongst patients and consumers in order to make money – rather unscrupulously in my view – from them.

Let us explore why the belief that "natural remedies" are without side effects is false. It would be useful at this stage to review Chapter 1 for a fuller understanding of what a "drug" is. For the rest of this discussion I shall assume that the reader understands a drug to be "a medicine or other substance which has a physiological effect when ingested or otherwise

---

[1] Willow Tree Image obtained from Wikimedia Commons under CC BY-SA 3.0 Ported Licence

introduced into the body." By this definition both "conventional medicines" and "natural remedies" are seen to be drugs since they modify the physiological behaviour of the body or are otherwise used to treat something affecting the body.

The way a lot of drugs work is that the active components mimic or block the effect of natural chemicals found in the body. This is often described in terms of a "lock and key" mechanism. As an example, the body naturally has what are referred to as "opiate receptors". When a person is in pain, the body naturally produces endorphins that stimulate these receptors and moderate the pain, otherwise it would be unbearable. It just so happens that the structure of molecules such as morphine is similar enough to these natural chemicals to be able to stimulate these receptors, sometimes more powerfully than the natural substance found in the body.

On the other hand, externally produced chemicals can bind to certain enzymes or structures and prevent normal physiological processes from occurring. This is the reasoning behind the use of certain drugs to prevent heartburn/indigestion and stomach ulcers though reducing the amount of acid in the stomach; or in depression through preventing the reuptake of what are regarded as "feel good" chemicals such as Serotonin.

This is of course a highly simplified explanation but it is accurate enough for our purposes.

There are exceptions to this. Emollients applied to the body to either hydrate it or prevent the skin drying out may not directly modify a specific physiological action, but we accept them as drugs anyway. Anaesthetics, which "numb" a local or produce general anaesthesia in major operations, also have a rather poorly understood mechanism of action. Again, certain drugs simply act by interacting with physical or chemical processes in the body. Antacids are a case in point. In some cases the mechanism remains unknown, even though the drugs are effective.

Finally, there are drugs that are primarily targeted not at the human body, but at pathogens affecting the human body. Known as antimicrobials (antibiotics, antifungals, antihelmitics and antivirals), these are designed to fight bacteria, fungi, protozoa and viruses by either destroying them or attenuating them to the point that the body can fight them itself. However, the body does recognise them as "foreign" with the result that they commonly elicit a physiological response from the body.

When you understand the above explanation, you begin to see that there is no difference between the way "natural products" work and the way medicines produced by industry work.

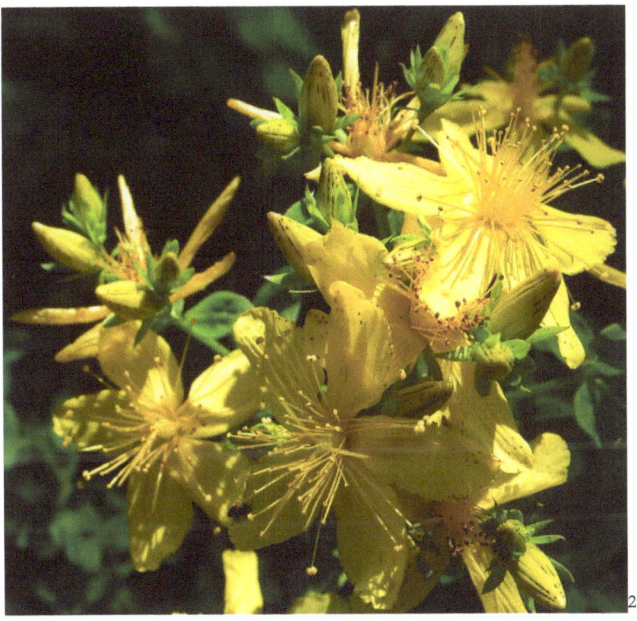

Figure 6 St John's Wort (Hypericum perforatum)

Take the example of St John's Wort, pictured above. Extracts from this are widely used as antidepressants or as mood enhancers by people that do

---

[2] St John's Wort Image obtained from Wikimedia Commons under CC BY-SA 3.0 Ported Licence

not wish to use "regular" antidepressants. The available evidence, however, points to its mechanism of action being similar to a combination of different types of antidepressants ((Butterweck, 2003: 17(8)).

Having mentioned the similarity of action between regular drugs and "natural remedies", it is also necessary to look at another misconception: the idea that natural products do not produce side effects.

"Side effects" normally arise from any of a number of potential causes:

1. As indicated above, drugs will mimic the action of natural body chemicals on certain receptors, enzymes or processes. Unfortunately, in the interests of efficiency, our bodies are designed in such a way that you can often find the same receptors, enzymes or processes at different parts of the body, in some cases performing different functions. When a drug is introduced into the body with the intention that it will affect one part, it might have unintended consequences at other parts as well. Take, for instance, the opiate drugs that we have referred to. They are effective in pain relief through actions on the central nervous system. However, since there are also opiate receptors in the gastrointestinal tract, the same drugs are dispersed via the blood street to these parts as well and tend to cause the unfortunate side effect of constipation through inhibiting gastrointestinal tract motility. Such side effects are arguably the most common.

2. There might be specific factors related to an individual that make that individual more prone to side effects. For instance, young children and the elderly are more likely to experience side effects due to differences in liver and kidney function or the way drugs are distributed in the body. Other differences, related to such factors as genes or race, mean that otherwise similar individuals respond to drugs differently.

3. Some people may actually react to the additional components used in the formulation, such as colorants, diluents or even preservatives.

4. Side effects do also arise from errors in dosing. When an individual takes too much of a drug, adverse effects are more likely to occur. This is illustrated on the diagram below and will be discussed in a later chapter.

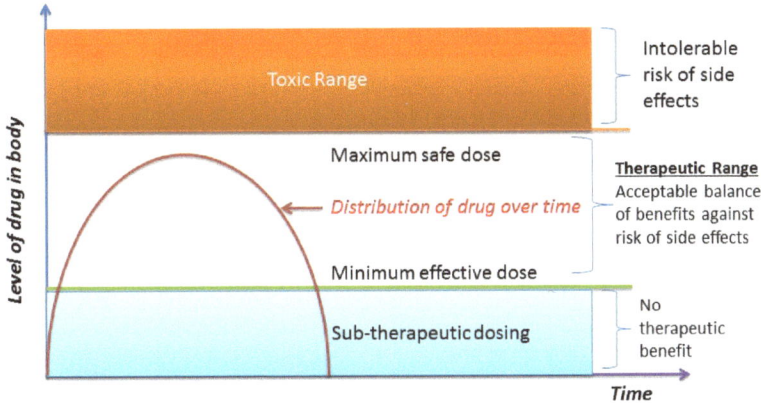

Figure 8 Dosing Decision Curve

Natural remedies are as prone to all of these as are regular medicines. In fact, it is possible to argue that standardised formulations are preferable to a lot of natural formulations and in fact reduce your likelihood of experiencing adverse effects for the following reasons:

1. Natural products do not come in "pure" form. A standard root or leaf contains several compounds, some of them with unknown properties and effects. It seems preferable in most cases to have a good idea what you are introducing into your body.

2. There is a lot of variability in the level of active component in different samples of the same natural product. If two people grow a batch of St John's Wort, not only are the final products from the two individuals likely to have different levels of the active components, different plants from each batch are likely to have concentrations as well. These will

have been influenced by the level of exposure to moisture, light or nutrients. A quantity that might have been safe in one sample might prove inadequate or toxic in another.

3. The safe therapeutic range, dose and dosing frequency will have been determined beforehand as a condition of granting a marketing licence for the product. This is not the case for a lot of natural products. When told to boil a raw root before consumption, in order to treat some medical condition, people often are not told how much water to use; how long to boil it for; or how long to keep the resultant solution.

Some people may feel that the arguments presented above are just theoretical and not based on real life observation. That is not true. There are texts, dedicated to natural products as medicines, that list the side effects to be expected from various products. In the United Kingdom, reliable information is available from the Pharmaceutical Press in the form of the publication simply entitled, "Herbal Medicines."

In addition to this, herbal medicines are known to interact not just with regular medicines taken concurrently, but potentially also with each other. It is useful at this point to highlight St. John's Wort as a common herbal medicines with a wide range of interactions and a strong need for monitoring by a health professional if being used with other medication. The Pharmaceutical Press publishes another volume, under the title, "Stockley's Herbal Drug Interaction," that is extremely useful as a reference tool for interactions involving the most common herbal medicines.

3: "Paracetamol (Acetaminophen) accumulates in the Human Body for Years"

There's an urban myth that has been circulating on the internet and e-mail inboxes since the year 2000 or so. It relates to Paracetamol and its supposed ability to accumulate in the body over a long time. One version of it is as follows:

"... When we were in Mumbai (India) a learned History professor there told us that the Parsees (A sect in India) used to take their Dead & lay them to rest at huge 'Wind Towers' (round structures that Look like Giant Water reservoirs, but open to the air). The Parsees never buried their dead, nor burned them. They leave them to the Birds of Prey (Vultures) to be eaten thus completing the Life Cycle..

Around 10 years ago, it was noticed that the Birds were dying off. Not many of them were left to consume the dead bodies (which started rotting away)...So, the Parsees had to change this mode of dealing with their dead... BUT, they wanted to know why a Custom that survived for hundreds of years had to be suspended?!!

They did Autopsies on Dead Birds (they were dying in huge #'s)..What was the Culprit??? PARACETAMOL (aka PANADOL).....!!

People started consuming pain-killers a decade ago, Panadol STAYS in the Liver for a Long Time...It ultimately accumulated in the Birds' systems & they couldn't cope with it!

Interesting to know..........

My husband was working in a hospital as an IT engineer, as the hospital is planning to set up a database of its patients and he knows some of the doctors quite well. The doctors used to tell him that whenever they have a headache, they are not willing to take PANADOL / PARACETAMOL. In fact, they will turn Herbal Medicine or find other alternatives. This is because Panadol is toxic to the body, and it harms the liver.

According to the doctor: 'Panadol will remain in the body for at least 5 years.....!!' And according to the doctor, there was an air-hostess who consumed lots of Panadol as she needed to stand all the time and work under lots of pressure. She's now in her early 30's, and she is undergoing kidney cleaning (DIALYSIS) every month.

Whenever we have a headache, that's because it is due to the electron/ion imbalance in the brain. Some alternative solution to cope with this matter is:

- *Drink lots of water.*

- *Another method will be to submerge your feet in a basin of warm water so that it brings the blood pressure down from your throbbing head.*

As Panadol is a pain killer, the more Panadol you take, the lesser would be your threshold for pain (your endurance level for pain). We all will fall ill as we age.

Imagine that we had spent our entire life popping quite a substantial amount of Panadol (Pain Killer), when you need to have a surgery or operation, you will need a much more amount of general anesthesia.

The thought is scary enough to turn me to Herbal Medicine or other healthier alternative. Value your health, value your life, THINK TWICE before you easily pop that familiar pill into your mouth again.

Please don't take too much PANADOL"

To start with there is some dodgy science in the e-mail, quoted above. The stuff about electron/ion imbalance is just plain wrong. The e-mail also seems to be a promotion for herbal medicines. That may be what the writer intended, but let us look at the validity of the main claim about the way the human body handles Paracetamol.

1. *The Allegation shows a Gross Misunderstanding of Paracetamol Metabolism*

Paracetamol, like every other food and chemical product that enters your body, has to pass through the liver at some point. The liver processes all the chemicals that your body takes in, ensuring that they are coupled with other chemicals to make them harmless/more soluble and eventually excreted. This process is referred to as metabolism. In the case of Paracetamol, there are three pathways involved in this, glucoronide conjugation, sulphate conjugation and – for a small proportion – a two-step process that involves hydroxylation followed by glutathione conjugation.

---

[3] Paracetamol Metabolism: Image courtesy of Wikipedia. Used under CC BY-SA 3.0

The by-products from the first two processes are harmless, but the intermediary product in the third stage (shown in red in the above diagram and referred to as NAPQI) is toxic and easily reacts with proteins in the liver cells leading to damage. This third process of getting rid of Paracetamol is generally called upon by the liver once the first two are saturated. However, it can itself get saturated pretty quickly once glutathione levels have been depleted, leading to an accumulation of the toxic intermediate metabolite (NAPQI), which then causes extensive liver damage. This is the basis for the recommended doses of Paracetamol: ensuring that the body does not build up levels of NAPQI to toxic levels. In the event that levels of NAPQI do rise to toxic levels, symptoms of toxicity appear within one to four days after an overdose. This is usually followed by a painful death unless other measures are adopted.

The main problem with the story above is that it alleges that Paracetamol would accumulate in the body over a period of five years; whereas we know that if you take the recommended dose at specified intervals, the standard metabolic processes outlined above would ensure that in about six hours the levels of Paracetamol in your system are close to negligible. It is not possible for anyone to accumulate the drug for more than a few days without dying.

2. The Genetic Variation Argument

It is known that differences between races sometimes mean that various enzymes are expressed at different levels between the races. A very common example is the low level of acetaldehyde dehydrogenase (sometimes referred to as alcohol dehydrogenase) among many people of Oriental descent, which leads to decreased tolerance of alcohol. This might lead to the allegation that the Indian Parsi people referred to above lack the "enzyme" responsible for the metabolism of Paracetamol. However, as indicated above, there are three main metabolic pathways involved in the metabolism of the drug. It is highly improbable that the population group would lack the enzymes responsible for all three metabolic processes. In addition, these metabolic processes are not created by the body specifically to metabolise Paracetamol. They naturally exist for a range of natural processes. Their absence would place the individual at serious risk of toxicity from other causes, not just Paracetamol intake.

3. The Numbers Don't Add Up

Assuming that both arguments above are flawed, and the Parsi people do indeed lack the hormones for metabolising Paracetamol, potentially leading to the accumulation of the drug in the system, then this leads to a further complication. It is known that the analgesic (pain-killing) effect of Paracetamol is attained when a dose (for the average adult) of between 500mg and 1000mg is taken. If the drug is not being excreted out of the body, then there is presumably no further need to take the drug and it may be assumed that the individuals would be content with just two tablets taken at very long intervals. There would be little added benefit from continued intake of the drug because its mechanism of action means that it has relatively mild analgesic effects. On this basis, any individual would have the equivalent of at most two tablets in his/her system at the point of death, and large numbers of individuals would need to be eaten by any individual vulture before it could build anything like the levels required for toxicity.

4. There are other more credible explanations

Available evidence suggests that there are at least three alternative feasible explanations for the decline in vulture numbers. The first of these is toxicity, albeit involving a different drug to Paracetamol. It appears that

Diclofenac, a non-steroidal anti-inflammatory drug, is a more likely culprit. Diclofenac is commonly used in animals as well as in humans. It is also known that Diclofenac and its metabolites can be toxic to some animals, particularly birds. This is the explanation accepted by the Royal Society for the Protection of Birds (RSPB). The following image shows a snapshot of the RSPB webpage dedicated to the problem.

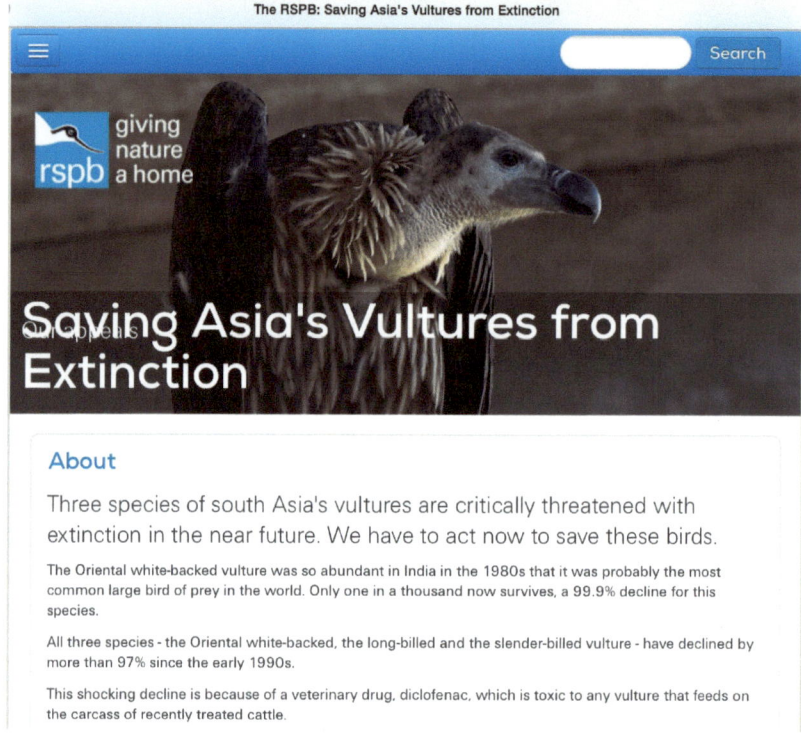

4

This also addresses the numbers conundrum. Vultures are indiscriminate eaters and will conceivably consume large numbers of dead animals treated with the drug, leading to accumulation of toxic quantities.

The other possible explanations relate to urbanisation and malaria. The former reduces breeding grounds and the latter is believed to kill the birds.

---

[4] View of www.rspb.org.uk webpage accessed September 2014.

The logical conclusion therefore, based on available reliable evidence, is that it is safe to continue taking Paracetamol within the recommended guidelines if there is a need to do so.

4: "The Flu Vaccine causes Flu"

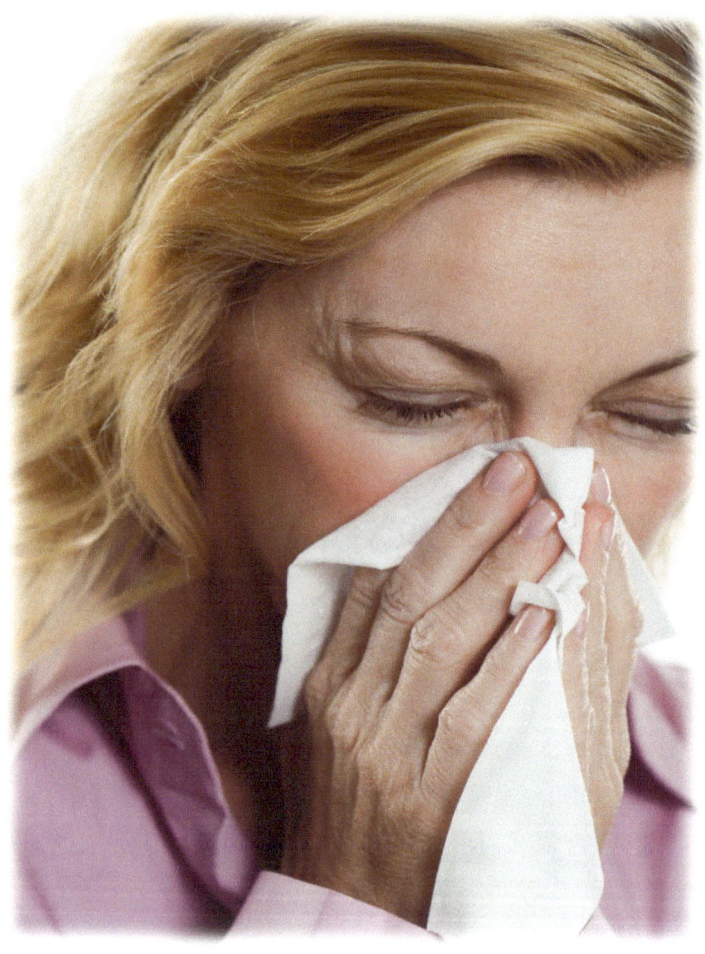

This is one of the more difficult myths to dispel. Most of the developed world advises that people in vulnerable groups get vaccinated against flu

---

[5] Image from Microsoft Clip Art

every year at the start of the flu season, which tends to be in autumn.

The people in the vulnerable groups are the elderly (i.e. over the age of 65), pregnant women and people with a range of medical conditions including the following:

- Heart conditions and complaints
- Chest complaints and breathing difficulties related to asthma, bronchitis and emphysema
- Serious kidney disease
- Low immunity due to medical conditions or treatments such as cancer or steroids
- Those that have had the spleen removed.

Health workers are also usually advised to get the flu vaccine because they are seen as posing a threat to vulnerable patient groups in the event that they develop "the flu". More details on this are available from the NHS Choices website.

The problem is that many people are convinced that if they get vaccinated, the vaccine itself will give them flu. This is often a result of previous experience with side effects of the flu vaccine, either in themselves or somebody they know. This is compounded by conspiracy theories over the safety of vaccines in general and the intentions of governments in allowing the licensing of vaccines.

The reality is that there is no singe effective licensed medicine that does not cause some side effects if some of the population. However, the overall benefits of the vaccine are greater that the risks. The Centres for Disease Control and Prevention (CDC) has the following to say regarding the question whether the flu vaccine causes flu:

Can the flu vaccine give me the flu?

"No, a flu vaccine cannot cause flu illness. Flu vaccines that are administered with a needle are currently made in two ways: the vaccine is made either with a) flu vaccine viruses that have been 'inactivated' and are therefore not infectious, or b) with no flu vaccine viruses at all (which is the case for recombinant influenza vaccine). The nasal spray flu vaccine does contain live viruses. However, the viruses are attenuated (weakened), and therefore cannot cause flu illness. The weakened viruses are cold-adapted, which means they are designed to only cause infection at the cooler temperatures found within the nose. The viruses cannot infect the lungs or other areas where warmer temperatures exist."

As indicated above, this does not mean that the flu vaccine does not cause side effects in at least part of the population some of the time. The CDC explains what the most common side effects are:

"While a flu vaccine cannot give you flu illness, there are different side effects that may be associated with getting a flu shot or a nasal spray flu vaccine. These side effects are mild and short-lasting, especially when compared to symptoms of bad case of flu.

The flu shot: The viruses in the flu shot are killed (inactivated), so you cannot get the flu from a flu shot. Some minor side effects that may occur are:

- Soreness, redness, or swelling where the shot was given,

- Fever (low grade),

- Aches

The nasal spray: The viruses in the nasal spray vaccine are weakened and do not cause severe symptoms often associated with influenza illness. In children, side effects from the nasal spray may include:

- Runny nose,

- Wheezing,

- Headache,

- Vomiting,

- Muscle aches,

- Fever

In adults, side effects from the nasal spray vaccine may include:

- Runny nose,

- Headache,

- Sore throat,

- Cough

If these problems occur, they begin soon after vaccination and are mild and short-lived."

Does this therefore mean that all the talk about problems with the flu vaccine is myth? Are there groups of people that cannot be given the vaccine for genuine medical reasons? The answer is, "Yes".

"Almost all people who receive influenza vaccine have no serious problems from it. However, on rare occasions, flu vaccination can cause serious problems, such as severe allergic reactions."

The reasons for this are normally predictable if the full medical history is known. There are classes of people that cannot be given the vaccine. Among these are babies below the age of six months and people with severe, life-threatening allergies to some of the components of the vaccine such as gelatin, antibiotics or eggs. It might be possible for those with egg allergies to still have the vaccine if this is done under the supervision of a specialist.

There are a number of other important considerations regarding the flu vaccine. To start with, it does not immediately offer protection from the flu and can take up to two weeks before it works. Secondly, the vaccine only offers protection against the predicted main types of flu for that season. If there is a difference between the strain that infects a person and what is in the vaccine, the vaccine offers reduced protection; although it must be stressed that the antibodies in the patient will still offer some protection. This means that it is still possible for a person that has had the vaccine to get flu.

Overall, the vaccine offers greater advantages than disadvantages for the following reasons:

1. It reduces the severity of the illness in people that have had the vaccine.

2. Where the strain in the vaccine matches the pandemic strain, the vaccine works i.e. it stops people getting flu

3. It helps protect vulnerable groups that are more susceptible to flu. These are listed at the beginning of this chapter.

4. It has been shown to significantly reduce hospitalizations and deaths from flu

5. It provides "head immunity". In other words, the more people there are that have had the vaccine, the less risk there is of a pandemic with resultant serious illness and death

If you still have any doubts, I strongly recommend you visit the NHS Choices (UK) or CDC (US) websites for more in-depth information.

5. "A Treatment is the same as a Cure"

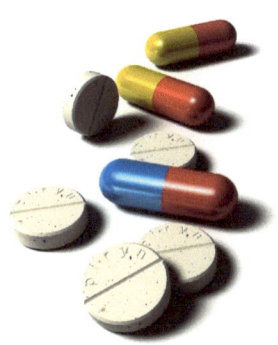

It's an average morning on a typical day and I'm talking to one of my patients. Mr. "Smith" has just been prescribed a new tablet for high blood pressure and he is apprehensive at taking a tablet every morning for the rest of his life.

"So, Mr Smith, do you understand why the doctor has given you this tablet?"

"I think so, son," he replies soberly. "I don't like tablets. I've never liked taking them. How long will I have to take these for? Is this a course?"

"I'm afraid it's a bit more complicated than that, Mr Smith," I reply. "Here, let me explain exactly why you need to keep taking these."

A short discussion on hypertension then follows; covering the mechanism of action of the drug in question and the benefits of treatment compared with the risks of non-compliance.

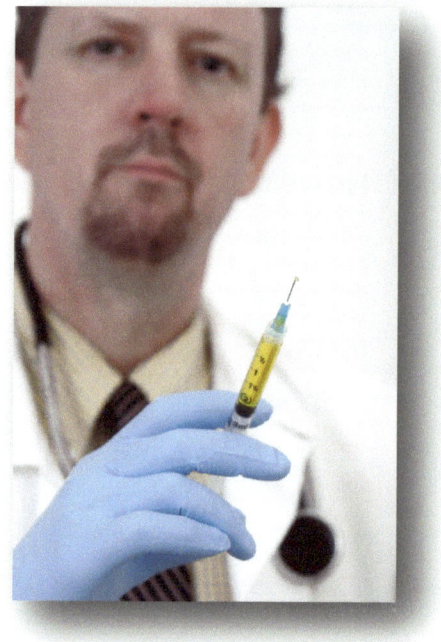

7

"Mr Smith" is an example of millions of people that believe that when you go to the doctor you always get a "cure" for whatever is wrong medically with you. My view of this is that it is wrong. The word "cure" suggests a restoration of health to a previous ideal state so that there is no need for further use of medication. For instance, many people in Mr Smith's position believe that if they are diagnosed with high blood pressure they only need to take tablets for a few months and then the high blood pressure is reversed so that they don't need to take medication any more.

---

[7] Image from Microsoft Clip Art

This, unfortunately, is not the case. In most cases people have to take these medicines for the rest of their lives.

Treatment, on the other hand, refers to bringing the symptoms of a disease or illness under control so as to enable the individual to live as normal a life as possible. What a doctor means when she says that she is treating your high blood pressure is that she will give you medication to bring down the blood pressure from unhealthy high levels to a level where they can be described as within the "normal" range. The medication works only as long as you keep taking it. "Treatment" thus refers to effectively managing symptoms of an illness rather than taking away illness altogether.

Is modern medicine capable of providing cures? Yes, in some cases it is. Quite often, however, the medicine/drug only keeps the symptoms under control and if the individual wants a "cure" in the absolute sense then this is only possible if that individual makes changes to his/her lifestyle that reverse what has brought on the illness, where this is possible. If the person is overweight, has high blood pressure and is taking medication for this (the treatment); then losing weight can reverse the high blood pressure and provide the cure (normal blood pressure).

In this, as in other cases where your doctor/pharmacist advises you to do so, it is important to keep taking the treatment until the cure arrives.

6: "Antidepressants are the only effective treatment for Depression"

It is important to understand that the solution to health problems does not always come in the form of a pill, tablet, liquid medicine, injection, cream or other formulation. This is true of both physical and mental illness. In the case of depression, this is especially important since current evidence suggests that the effectiveness of antidepressants varies according to the severity of depression and the actual condition being treated.

For those that have missed the debate around antidepressants, what we currently know about antidepressants is that they are more likely to work for severe depression than for mild forms. In addition, recent studies indicate that antidepressants work for between 50 and 65 per cent of patients, compared with about 25 to 30 per cent improvement for people taking dummy pills (placebos).[8] Some people argue that this means that in real terms antidepressants work for around a third of people for whom they are prescribed.

---

[8] Figures accepted by both the Royal College of Physicians and NHS Choices as reflected on the respective websites in September 2014.

So what are the alternatives?

Both the charity Mind UK and the Scottish Intercollegiate Guidelines Network (SIGN) provide some useful information on non-drug approaches to treating depression. The information can be summarised as follows:

There are three types of recommended non-drug approaches to the treatment of depression:

1.   Psychological Therapies.

These include the following:

- Behavioural Activation;
- Individual Cognitive Behavioural Therapy (CBT);
- Couple-focused therapy where the relationship is relevant to the condition;
- Interpersonal Therapy;
- Mindfulness-based Cognitive Therapy in groups;
- Problem Solving Therapy;
- Short Term Psychodynamic Therapy

2.   Self-Help.

This may include the following:

- Guided self-help based on CBT/behavioural principles;
- Computerised CBT within the context of self-help

3.   Structured Exercise

As with standard drug therapy, it is crucial that those responsible for providing these alternative treatments be competent in doing so; something reflected in the SIGN statement that *"practitioners delivering psychological therapies"* … should … *"be trained to approved levels of competency, participate in continuing professional development and be registered with the appropriate governing body. They should be receiving on-going supervision."*

There are also some popular approaches for which there is insufficient evidence to warrant recommending as treatment. These include:

1. Counselling

2. Family Therapy

3. Hypnotherapy

4. Music Therapy

5. Reminiscence Therapy and a range of other services

6. Use of herbal and nutritional supplements such as folate, inositol, polyunsaturated fatty acids, S-adenosyl-L-methionine, chromium, ginseng, ginkgo biloda, glutamine or selenium

7. Complementary and alternative therapies such as acupuncture, animal-assisted therapy, homeopathy, light therapy, massage therapy, yoga

When it come to the popular St. John's Wort, the guidelines advice against it and actually give the following recommendations: *"Healthcare professionals should not advise use of extract of Hypericum (St John's wort) for patients with depression due to the lack of standardisation of dose and the risk of interactions with several common medications including the contraceptive pill. Where individual patients are using extract of Hypericum (St John's wort) for treatment of depression, the general practitioner should facilitate full consideration of potential drug interactions."*

7: "If You Live Right, You Will Never have to take any Medication in Your Life"

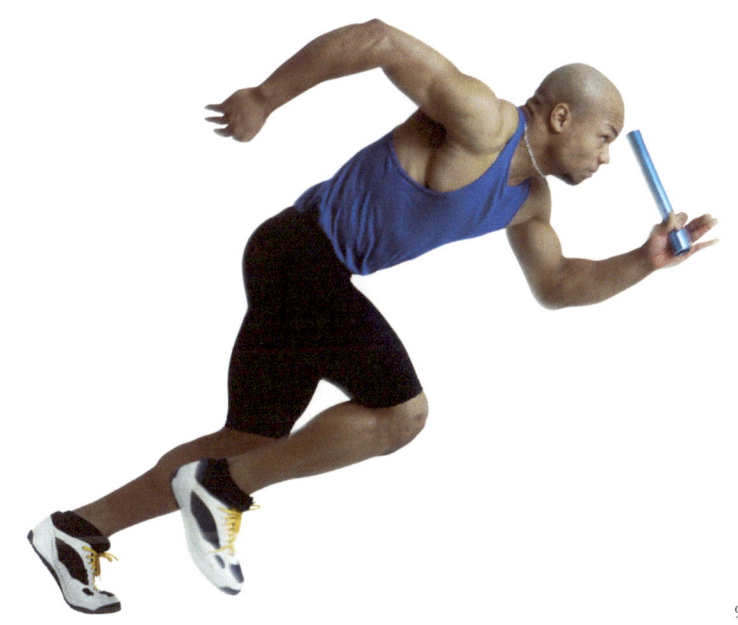

9

We live in an age in which people have learnt that a lot of illnesses are caused by lifestyle choices. The causes of common conditions such as high blood pressure, Type 2 diabetes, high cholesterol levels in the blood and a lot of cancers can be traced to choices around food, smoking and exercise. Infective diseases such as venereal diseases can also often be traced to unwise lifestyle choices.

---

[9] Athlete image from Microsoft Clip Art

The problem arises when people assume that all illness is a result of poor personal choices and thus avoidable. This is not true. We live in an imperfect world and some imperfections affect our bodies as well. Some illnesses are a result of factors beyond an individual's control.

Take for example, conditions that arise from infections. Influenza (the 'flu') tends to attack the human population with predictable regularity. As discussed above, the use of the vaccine, or indeed symptomatic management once an individual gets the flu or even a common cold, can greatly reduce the discomfort normally associated with infection. We can also be exposed to a variety of pathogens via the environment, animal and human hosts. Few people would argue against the use of prophylactic drugs when travelling to an area with a high risk of malaria. Similarly, fewer still would argue against the use of appropriate medication if exposed to and infected by deadly conditions such as tuberculosis or Ebola; for which no amount of lifestyle measures would prove adequate in effecting a cure.

It is also known that there is a genetic link to conditions such as asthma, eczema, high blood pressure, high cholesterol levels or endometriosis among many others. If you happen to be have such genes, then you are much more likely to have to take medication to mitigate against the effect of such genetic predispositions. That is why you often find that the children of parents with asthma need to start using inhalers at an early age; despite not having had a chance to make any personal lifestyle choices that might influence this outcome.

Again, it is likely that if you are of Asian descent (Indian/Pakistani); you might find that you are more likely to have elevated cholesterol levels that increase your cardiovascular risk. Regarding this point, further studies are needed to determine whether a radical change of lifestyle factors, including diet, reduces the risk to a level comparable to that of other populations groups.

It is also generally accepted that as we grow older then more things are likely to go wrong. The body gets to a point where it is not as efficient in repairing itself, stopping uncontrolled cell growth and getting rid of such things as free radicals that are believed to be a factor in the development of some cancers. That is why a lot of clinicians believe that in the absence of other causes, everyone would probably get cancer if they lived long enough.

There are of course proven ways of reducing the likelihood of having to take medication. These include regular exercise, get adequate sleep, maintain an ideal body weight, eating a healthy diet, effectively managing stress levels and even maintaining healthy social and spiritual influences, as has been confirmed by various studies. The important point to bear in mind is that whilst these are very effective, it is important to maintain regular contact with medical personnel and to be aware that there might arise an occasional need to take some form of medication.

8: "There is a formal category of drugs referred to as 'legal highs'"

In the past several years there have been numerous unfortunate deaths of mainly young people due to what have now become popularly known as 'legal highs'. The death of just one person is an enormous tragedy and I do not wish to trivialise any of these deaths in any way. My problem is with the presentation of the cause in some of the popular press and media outlets. Take the following recent article from a major paper:

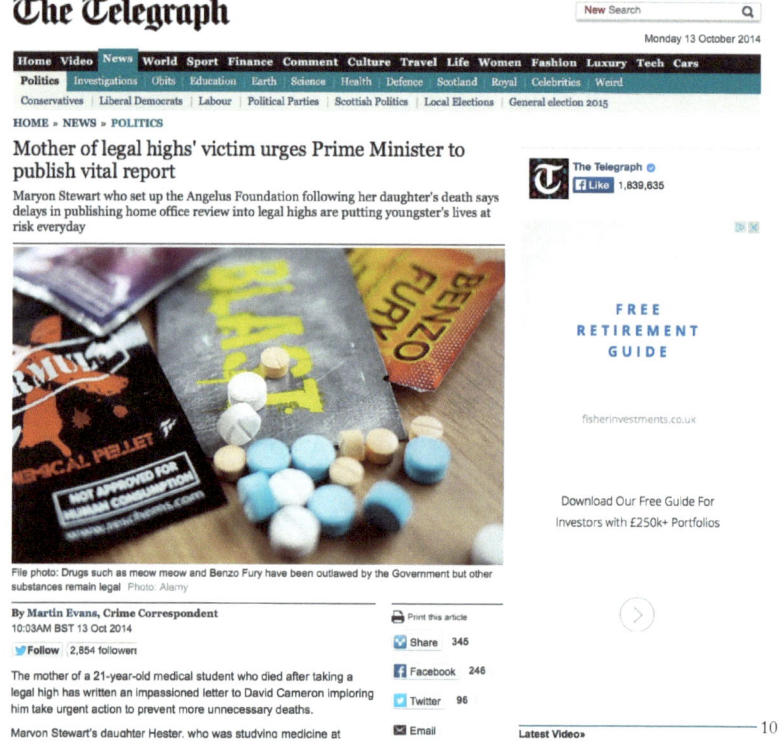

---

[10] Page accessed via Telegraph website (www.telegraph.co.uk), 12 October, 2014

The typical story follows a familiar pattern:

1. A naïve/innocent young person went to a party
2. The young person was given a drug with or without alcohol to enhance the experience
3. The drug was "legal"
4. The drug turned out to be lethal for the young person
5. The government knew/or should have known, that the drug was widely available and popular on the club and party scenes
6. The government knew/should have known that the drug was potentially lethal
7. The government should have outlawed the drug
8. The government is therefore at fault

Let us focus on the third point above as it has a bearing on the rest of the arguments. The term "legal" needs to be defined. It can mean one of two things:

1. That something has been specifically defined as permissible or mandatory in the law of the land. Hence it is legal for a mature man and woman – who are not close relatives or still married to other people – to seek to get married via the usual channels.

2. That something has not yet been defined as breaching any existing laws and so can be done without legal consequence until the law is changed to forbid it.

A lot of people speak about "legal" party drugs as if they belong to the former category. In reality they belong to the second category. With the obvious exceptions of alcohol and tobacco – and to a lesser extent marijuana – most governments are reluctant to license new drugs for recreational use. Our understanding of health has improved to such an extent that the risks associated with recreational drug use are known to outweigh the benefits.

In the UK, drugs and medicines for human use generally fall into three category with respect to availability for supply to the public. These are prescription-only medicines (POMs), General Sales List (GSL) medicines and an in-between category that can only be obtained from pharmacies (P Medicines). These drugs undergo rigorous testing processes for safety and appropriate dosing before being granted marketing authorisations (i.e. the right to be sold). Drugs used recreationally in clubs and at parties to induce feelings of euphoria or relaxation are not in any of these categories.

Such "recreational products" tend to be available on account of three main reasons:

1. Drugs and chemicals may have legitimate uses for humans, animals or plants and then someone discovers their euphoric or hallucinogenic properties and starts to market them outside the licensed indication as raves and clubs. Ketamine, an anaesthetic, probably falls into this category. So does mephedrone.

2. People may divert a known (legal) psychoactive compound onto the club scene because of its popularity.

3. A new psychoactive compound might be synthesized either from scratch or by modifying existing licensed products. Crystal meth, which can be synthesized from pseudoephedrine that is available from pharmacies over the counter, is an example of this.

In most cases the development of the new drug and its availability on the club scene outpace the law. The law is also often hamstrung by the need to have a robust evidence base for decisions made on drug categorization. Hence, if there is a new recreational "drug" available on the club scene, it will not have under undergone rigorous testing beforehand, its potential side effects will not be fully known and the "government" might not even be aware of its availability.

That being the case, it is perhaps expecting a lot of the legal authorities to be able instantaneously capable of declaring every potentially dangerous product illegal. At the same time, the fact that a product is not on the "naughty list" should not form the basis for decision-making on whether to use it or not. Education on this is crucial. Perhaps we need to have a debate on why, as a society, we need to use recreational chemicals to enhance our enjoyment of social events. Although the horse has truly bolted and fled with respect to alcohol and tobacco, we have a chance to stem the tide when it comes to other drugs.

9: "The link between the MMR vaccine and Autism ... "

This book would not be complete without a discussion of one of the most elaborate medical frauds of the past century, the repercussions of which we still suffer today.

In 1998 Doctor Andrew Wakefield published a paper in the *Lancet* in which he claimed to show a link between the administration of the MMR vaccine and the development of autism and bowel disease. His research and conclusions were subsequently proven to be false, yet they caused a massive decline in the uptake of the vaccine in the UK and North America. They also fed into conspiracy theories of government cover-ups and malicious intent by governing authorities.

The truth is that there remains no proven link between the MMR vaccine and autism. No independent researchers have been able to reproduce the results claimed by Andrew Wakefield. He has now been struck off the register of medical practitioners maintained by the General Medical Council (GMC) The sad reality is that he remains unrepentant and continues to make money in the United States from speaking engagements related to his initial discredited publications.

Andrew Wakefield put many children at risk unnecessarily; now known to have been done out of selfish interest. Thanks to the investigative work of Brian Deer[11], working for Channel 4 and the Sunday Times, the

---

[11] http://www.briandeer.com

motivations and methods behind the work of Andrew Wakefield were laid bare for the world to see. Among the many findings were the following:

1. Andrew Wakefield was shown to have financial conflict of interest in the studies. While denouncing the so-called dangers of the MMR jab, he was secretly involved in steps to register an alternative single measles vaccine from which he stood to gain financially. He had actually applied for a patent for this before publishing his work on MMR. In addition to this he was planning to release a diagnostic kit based on his findings.

2. He subjected the children to unnecessary invasive medical procedures such as colonoscopies and lumbar punctures.

3. He was responsible for many children getting measles; as the parents read the claims he had made and that were publicised by the press.

4. He failed to get the necessary consent from parents, carers and ethics committees for the studies.

5. He was shown to have been under contract with solicitors whose intent was to eventually sue the manufacturers of the MMR vaccine.

6. He was convicted of dishonesty and abuse of mentally challenged children and his work was subsequently described as an 'elaborate fraud' in the British Medical Journal (BMJ) in 2011[12]. The BMJ notes that he deliberated falsified data towards nefarious ends.

7. The Lancet has since retracted the initial paper that Doctor Wakefield had submitted in 1998.

While it is true that most parents of children with autism are motivated by a desire to find out if there is an identifiable cause for the condition, available evidence suggests that a significant number of people that have

---

[12] Godlee F, Smith J, Marcovitch H (2011). "Wakefield's article linking MMR vaccine and autism was fraudulent". *BMJ* **342**: c7452. doi:10.1136/bmj.c7452. PMID 21209060.

promoted the link between autism and MMR have often been driven by the objective to eventually sue the manufacturers and/or the government.

Both the Sunday Times of 12 October, 2014[13]; and Brian Deer[14] on his website report the court case of a mother that had gone to extensive dishonest lengths to try to prove a link between her son's autism and the MMR vaccine. In his evaluation of the case the judge, Mr Justice Baker, concluded that the mother had lied about her son's adverse reactions to the vaccine. Brian Deer notes that this is something he has observed in other cases, parents lying in compensation cases over MMR. In this case there was a connection between the mother in the court case and Andrew Wakefield in that the woman was one of several women that had come together on the basis of Wakefield's publications with the intention of suing the manufacturers. More details are available on Brian Deer's website.

None of this is intended to demonise the poor mothers of children with autism. As indicated, the belief of a link between autism and MMR is founded on faulty logic and evidence. Perhaps the last word on this should be given to the Sunday Times piece from the 12th of October, 2014:

"Here was a mother condemned like few others. It shows how Wakefield's shadow continues to fall long after he was struck off. For E could be countless mothers, particularly in America where hardly a month passes without an appearance by Wakefield at conferences crowded with mother warriors. They trust him, I think, because the alternative is to blame themselves for their children's condition.

The truth, of course, is that nobody is to blame and all deserve compassion, not fuel for their anguish."

---

[13] http://briandeer.com/solved/st-october-12-2014-lying-mother.htm
[14] http://briandeer.com/solved/mother-lied-protection-mmr-1.htm

10. "You Need to Stock Up on Medication before a Bank Holiday"

This one is a major problem that all pharmacies face just before any bank holiday (known as public holiday in some countries). It feels like the majority of patients panic and want to have a full month's supply of all their medicines in the house, "just in case". This is surprising when you consider that the typical pharmacy is never closed for more than an extra two days at a time for bank holidays; these two days being Christmas and Boxing day.

Perhaps the best way to express the impressions of a lot of pharmacy teams is in the form of an imaginary letter written by a pharmacist to a patient just before Christmas.

"Dear Patient

First of all I wish to express my gratitude to you for providing me with a means to make a living. It is true that I went into this profession because I genuinely wanted to help people who had fallen ill. I thought it important for me to combine my interest in science with something beneficial for society as a whole and so I chose something that offered the chance to make a meaningful impact on people's lives. I genuinely look forward to those encounters when you ask me about medicines or the symptoms that your or your loved one are experiencing; so that I have the chance to improve your quality of life. I get immense satisfaction from seeing you a couple of weeks later looking better.

I hope by now that you have realized that I am not just interested in flogging a bottle of medicine in order to make a quick profit. I will often refuse to make a sale even if it hurts my bottom line; all because I think it is much more important that you get the right treatment and not merely what you or the internet think you need at that time.

Believe me it's not as easy or pleasant a decision to make as it sounds. I have profit targets to meet and superiors to report to. I have ethical obligations to sell to you only what I know to have a sound evidence base for clinical effectiveness, even when you believe that the medicine advertised on TV is the wonder portion to solve your very problem. I sadly don't have a say on everything stocked at the premises in which I work and so you may find that I do not readily recommend everything you wish to buy, especially those portions of water in small bottles and with fancy names; or many of the cough mixtures that thousands swear by; or even the tablets for cold that you also find at the local garage. Powers higher that I am are trying to sort out this mess at national government level but I do not see much of a solution in the near future.

Despite all this, I like to think that our relationship is broadly positive. I do my best to get your repeat medicines ready ahead of time if you are on any of our managed prescription repeat schemes. When you bring your own prescription I try to get it ready for you as quickly as possible and I aim to make time for a decent chat with you about your medicines once a year or so. If you have a new medicine I definitely make time for you as it's important that I check that you know how to use it, have the right level of support and that it works well with your other medication.

Having said this, there's just one teeny wincey thing that puzzles me. Every year around this time you seem to panic at the thought that the pharmacy will be closed over the Christmas holidays. I would understand if pharmacies did what some industries do: shut down for a couple of weeks over the festive season. However, we are only closed just for two days (Christmas and Boxing Day) in the first week and one day (New Year's Day) the following week. In fact, it is quite likely that a pharmacy not too far from you is on a holiday rota and will be open on at least one of those days; not to mention your average supermarket pharmacy that will probably be open on Boxing Day. This means that, logically, your access to our health services described above should not be compromised. In theory the closures should only affect a small number of patients whose repeats are due on the three days on which we are closed. However, since we generally have excellent arrangements with our local surgeries to get your prescriptions done a few days before they are actually due, I expect that the even such patients should be able to pick up their medicines from the pharmacy a few days early without a big impact on the pharmacy operations.

As it is the opposite is true. The same internal forces that cause us to go overboard with our shopping even for ordinary food seem to influence our outlook on medicines. You would not get a more panicked response if you put a sign up at pharmacies that read,

"The world is coming to an end on Christmas Eve. Get your prescription medicines and stock up!"

Perhaps there's a part of our brains that's wired like animals that hibernate in winter: only they store their food in their bodies and sleep though the cold; while we feel the need to stock up on food and medicines in our pantries and cupboards.

What are the risks associated with doing so? Well, for a start medicines are not like food. If you have too many of them around the house you raise the risk that they will fall into the wrong hands and be taken by somebody else. This can have severe consequences if that person is a child, is allergic to them, is on other medicines that interact or has an underlying condition whose symptoms are worsened by taking these medicines. As you might well appreciate, death could be the unfortunate consequence of inappropriate intake of your medicine in this situation.

Secondly it increases the risk of waste and loss. With too many medicines around the house some might get "misplaced" and so cause your tablets to go "out of sync", thus creating the need for you to order them early. Eventually you find that you accumulate more of one type than the others and have to dispose of the excess. I see this with depressing regularity and my heart bleeds at the value of money that we have to dispose of in the form of patient-returned drugs.

Thirdly it raises the risk that you make the medicines less clinically effective because of poor storage. Pharmacies have a legal duty to keep medicines under special temperature, humidity and light conditions. This is not always possible in a normal house.

Where do you keep your medicines? If you keep them in the bathroom then it is possible that the moisture levels are too high; if in the kitchen *in a drawer/ unit by the hob then both temperature and moisture might be a concern; if in the fridge then you not only worry about the level of access for children but also the extent to which you can guarantee that the temperature will be kept between 2^OC and 8^OC despite several people opening the fridge door to get food and drinks over a period of many weeks. Of course if you keep them in the bedroom then you need to make sure they are "out of sight and reach of children". Light, temperature and moisture can all have a dramatic effect on the stability of medicines. Incorrect levels can lead to medicines losing their potency and thus not being as effective as their nominal label strength indicates.*

So, what am I saying about your medicines and the Christmas period? If you check your medicines and find that you have enough for the next three weeks, then you are sorted and there is no need to panic. You have enough to last you into next year. Just follow your standard reordering schedule for your next repeat, allowing a week or so between the request and when you can pick up your medicines from the pharmacy.

If you are running out in the next week or so and have signed up to your preferred pharmacy's managed repeat scheme, in all probability the pharmacy has either already ordered your next repeat or will do so soon. Call the pharmacy at least five days before you run out to confirm that your prescription will be in by the due date. If you have not signed up then now is a good time to put in your request at your surgery.

Finally, if you are one of the few whose next repeat actually falls on the holiday dates then call your pharmacy at least five working days beforehand to make sure that the prescription is being sorted. Our least favourite patients are those that come in just before closing time on

Christmas Eve or New Years' Eve with a request for an emergency supply "to cover the holidays". There's a small legal minefield there that I'd love to discuss if I could make the time. Putting us under pressure on the Eves of the holidays increases the risk of us making dispensing errors. Remember, we do not wish to cause harm by issuing a wrong drug or giving wrong directions as a result of what could be seen as avoidable pressure.

I trust you will give my letter full and appropriate consideration.

Yours faithfully

Your Pharmacist

11. "Miscellaneous Myths"

This section has shorter myths that should be relatively quick to go through. Although some are shorter than others, overall they are an average of one page long.

"Doctors know everything about health and drugs"

Some patients expect their doctor to immediately be able to tell them everything about the medicines they are taking and the medical conditions they suffer from. They express surprise that their family doctor does not know everything to do with health and has to look up things or refer certain cases to specialists.

The question they ask is, "Well, did you not study the whole human body at medical school? In that case you should be able to figure out what's wrong with me."

The reality is that even the long years that a family doctor spends learning and practising medicine do not guarantee that she/he becomes the omniscient repository of all medical information. Doctors have finite capabilities, as do all human beings.

Nurses, physiotherapists, radiographers, dentist and pharmacists all have unique sets of skills that doctors do not have, but which help ensure more rounded care for patients.

"Dr. Google® will always have the right answer"

For some patients it appears that if something has been published on the internet, then it must be true and, in addition, it must apply to their own individual experience. The need for critical analysis in reviewing the source of any information is lost on some individuals; as is the small but not insignificant truth that a few minutes/hours on the internet do not grant you the diagnostic and prescribing powers that take the average doctor several years of learning and practice to acquire.

There is also the need to have the requisite background knowledge in order to evaluate the accuracy of any information available on the web. The reason there are disclaimers on all health information websites and online forums is that the publishers wish to protect themselves against the hazards on such inappropriate use of the information published. So, while it is important to take ownership of your own health, don't assume that what you have read or watched on the internet is the final word on the issue. Sometimes checking information on the internet is like gambling: you could win some, but if you lose, you lose big time!

"There should not be a delay in getting my medication ready. It's only tablets!"

This one irks all professionals, but pharmacists more so than others. It not only shows impatience, but creates the impression that medication is no different to food or other consumer items. Pharmacists use clinical skills in evaluating the suitability of a prescription for the patient's condition, the accuracy of the dose, the possibility of interaction with other medication, the potential for side effects and the overall known factors about the patient's state of health. There are increased risks in rushing through the process of dispensing any prescriptions as this may lead to errors and unpleasant health consequences for the patient affected, hence the pharmacists are not usually impressed at this comment.

The misconception about the time required to prepare medication at a pharmacy is often, but not always, associated with a belief that one can "speed along" the process by having a taxi waiting outside. Not only does this show a lack of knowledge of the checks required as part of the dispensing process (as discussed above), it suggest that the patient views his own condition as more pressing than those of everyone else in the pharmacy. The comment made by one pharmacist was, "It surprises me how patients will sit patiently for an hour or two at the surgery, yet when they come to the pharmacy they cannot even wait for fifteen minutes for their prescriptions to be processed."

"The doctor automatically sends the prescription to the pharmacy every month"

This is a problem faced by pharmacists and doctors alike. It arises when patients have a misunderstanding of the process involved in reordering their medication ("repeat prescriptions" as they are known in the UK or "refills" as they are known in North America). Some patients expect to just walk into a pharmacy when their medication has run out and get a new supply for the following month without having made any arrangements for supply of the repeat; either through reordering it themselves or through a pre-existing arrangement with the pharmacy to undertake this.

One receptionist, exasperated at yet another such demand from a patient, firmly retorted to the patient,

"Mr Jones! We have thousands of patients at this practice, and we serve hundreds of them daily. You seriously do not expect that in the course of my job I will remember that one patient – You! – has not ordered his medication on a particular day of the month! That is just unreasonable!"

"There is a treatment in tablet/capsule/injection form for every illness under the sun"

There are a surprisingly large number of patients that think that the solution to every health problem lies in a bottle or in tablet form. This is plainly not true when it comes to "lifestyle" diseases such as obesity, hypertension, type 2 diabetes or smoking related illnesses. In such cases the most effective solutions – at least in the initial stages - lie in making relatively simple changes to the lifestyle: increasing exercise to recommended levels, cutting down on alcohol, quitting smoking and having healthy eating habits, among other healthy lifestyle choices. Patients are however often unwilling to forego their preferred vice and think that the solution will come in a convenient dosage form without their having to give up what they know is unhealthy for them. Naturally such hopes are never realised in practice.

"All antibiotics interact with contraceptives, making them ineffective."

In the past it was believed that broad spectrum antibiotics interfered with entero-hepatic to such a significant extent that those taking oral contraceptives had to use additional barrier contraception. This has now been shown not to be the case. Additional contraception is not required unless:

- The antibiotic is a proven hepatic enzyme inducer (Rifampicin and Rifabutin are quick examples that come to mind)
- The woman experiences diarrhoea as a result of taking the antibiotics
- Vomiting is experienced as a result

"The Health Professional always knows more than the Patient"

A study published in the British Medical Journal in November 2013 debunked this myth. By looking at the experiences of diabetic patients that had received additional education about their condition, the study made the following observations:

"... *interactions within the health system following patient education could be fraught. Participants emerged from the course with greater condition-specific knowledge than many of the healthcare professionals they encountered. When these professionals did not understand what their patients were trying to do and were uncomfortable trusting their expertise, there could be serious consequences for these patients' ability to continue effective self-management.*"

It concluded as follows:

"*Patients who have in-depth knowledge of their condition encounter problems when their expertise is seen as inappropriate in standard healthcare interactions, and expertise taught to patients in one branch of medicine can be considered non-compliant by those who are not specialists in that field. Although patient education can give people confidence in their own self-management skills, it cannot solve the power imbalance that remains when a generalist healthcare professional, however well meaning, blocks access to medication and supplies needed to manage chronic diseases successfully. There is a role for those involved in primary and hospital care, including those supporting and training healthcare professionals, to recognise these problems and find ways to acknowledge and respect chronic patients' biomedical and practical expertise.*"

"More and Stronger is Always Better"

There is sometimes the temptation to believe that if so much of a drug is effective enough in reducing pain or controlling an infection, then increasing the dose will be even more effective and might quickly eliminate the infection if that happens to be the problem. The reality is that this reasoning is often flawed. If you have read the earlier chapter on herbal medicines and side effects you will have come across the dose response curve below.

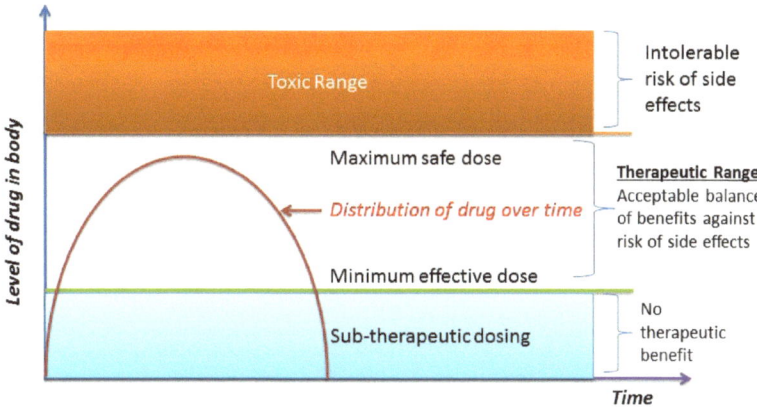

From the curve we can learn a few things about dosing with drugs:

1. Drugs have a safe "therapeutic range' within which the balance between effectiveness and adverse effects has been optimised. Taking more than the recommended range increases the likelihood of experiencing side effects. This is discussed in greater detail in Chapter 2.

2. It is actually possible that there might be no more additional benefits to be gained from taking the drug. Drugs can reach a peak 'effective dose' beyond which there are practically no benefits from additional doses; although side effects will continue to increase.

3. The unnecessary doses are effectively wasted even if the side effects are tolerable. This is not something we would wish to encourage.

"Water tablets are for those that have difficulty going to the loo"

Among the many things that pharmacists do is the job of trying to simplify medical terminology and the mechanisms of action of drugs so that these are easily understood by patients. For instance, patients on aspirin are often aware that the 'baby aspirin' helps to "thin the blood' in order to prevent 'heart attacks'. Similarly, patients on inhalers are usually trained to recognise the brown inhaler as the "preventer" and the blue one as the "reliever". Such simplifications are usually helpful in improving the patients' understanding of their medication and in improving compliance.

There are situations, however, when the 'simplifications' introduce further complications. An example is the class of drugs known as diuretics. These are often referred to as "water tablets". I had come to accept the loose redefinition until recently when a chance conversation with a patient showed a serious misunderstanding of their role.

I had started listing all her drugs and their functions when I got to the diuretic and decided to say it was a "water tablet'.

"What?" was the surprised response. "I'm not on a water tablet."

I started to explain that the tablet in question belonged to the class of tablets normally referred to as water tablets; something about which she was markedly unimpressed.

'My doctor hasn't told me that I'm on a water tablet. Water tablets are for people that have problems going to the toilet. I don't have any such problems," she said wryly.

I then had to take some time to clear her confusion.

The fact is that we have adopted the term 'water tablets' simply because diuretics, by nature, work on the kidneys to increase the amount of urine (hence water) being excreted from the body. This is seen as of value in the following situations:

1.   It reduces the volume of liquid (plasma) in the circulatory system, thus reducing the workload on the heart and reducing the blood pressure as a result.

2.   Where there is accumulation of liquid (oedema) in the lungs or other part of the body due to heart failure (or failure of one part of the heart), they help the body get rid of the accumulated liquid.

As can be seen, the diuretics are not used to make up for a patient's compromised kidney function. In fact, where renal function is severely compromised many of them cannot be used at all. Further information on this is available from your pharmacist or doctor.

"If it's green and phlegmy, then it's a sign that you need antibiotics."

If you've followed medical news over the past few years, you will be aware of the antibiotic crisis looming over our heads as human beings. The discovery of penicillin and other antibiotics brought in a golden era of survival for the human race. In the past, people's lives were decimated by microbes. However, antibiotics ushered in a new era of survival and longevity. Sadly, the lethal bugs have found ways to evade the devastation caused by antibiotics and the golden age for human survival is at risk.

Part of the reason for antibiotic resistance in microbes is the inappropriate prescribing of antibiotics. This happens, for instance, when people have a cough or cold and start producing green phlegm. For many this is an indication that they have an infection that needs antibiotics.

This is usually not the case. When you have a cold, your body sends white blood cells to your nose and chest. These cells release enzymes to kill the infection – and might themselves die in the line of duty as well. The dead invading cells, with the enzymes and fallen body soldiers, coagulate into that greenish, phlegmy mucus that your body understandably wants to get rid of when you cough. Antibiotics are often of no value in this situation because colds are of viral origin anyway.

It helps to be aware that you can have clear mucus and have a serious underlying infection; and that at times the mucus might have a brownish or reddish tinge from blood. It is important to consider these in the context of other symptoms such as pain, fever, severity, duration, location on the body and other relevant personal or societal factors. (If there is an epidemic of an infectious disease, for example, you are probably better off erring on the side of caution.) If you are in doubt, ask your pharmacist, NHS direct (in the UK) or call your doctor.

"Taking lots of medication is an unavoidable part of growing old."

This might seem like a contradiction of the arguments earlier about the maintenance of good lifestyle habits as not being a guarantee of never having to take medication. It is not.

We have come to accept that with the onset of old age comes a raft of illnesses such as Alzheimer's (including dementia), hypertension, diabetes or even cancer. However, several studies have blown this understanding to smithereens. It is true that a lot of people spend the last few decades (and increasingly longer) of their lives slowly dying and sustained by medication. However, the understanding is now firmly established that a lot of this is avoidable if people make appropriate lifestyle choices at all stages of their lives, especially in youth.

In November 2005 National Geographic published the outcome of studies it had undertaken on longevity and quality of life into old age.[15] It identified three distinct groups of people across the world that enjoyed both. These were the residents of Okinawa, Sadinia and Loma Linda (Carlifonia). Discounting genetic factors, the studies showed that appropriate lifestyle choices and habits can greatly enhance the likelihood a healthy life up to a century or more, relatively free from the aches, pains and diseases that typically attend old age.

---

[15] http://ngm.nationalgeographic.com/2005/11/longevity-secrets/buettner-text

The habits that were identified as crucial for the attainment of such a life were the following[16]:

1. Conscious choices to reduce stress levels, particularly among men.

2. Strong social 'family-style' bonding. This need not be immediate family members but could be due to strong links such as are offered by a vibrant religious community (church in the case of the Loma Linda group) or a group of long-term friends.

3. Eating a diet that's as close to natural as possible, free from processed foods. This is enhanced by having a largely plant-based diet; with a balanced vegetarian diet being a notably positive option.

4. Getting regular, adequate exercise and avoiding a sedentary lifestyle. Such a lifestyle includes exposure to clean air and sunshine.

5. Having a reason/belief beyond the immediate for waking up. This might be in the form of a strong religious belief and/or transcendent culture.

6. Abstinence from cigarettes, alcohol or other stimulants; aided by adequate intake of clean water.

7. Having a weekly day of rest to completely unplug from normal daily activity; otherwise known as the Sabbath.

If you wish to find out more you can view the video yourself at the link indicated below.

---

[16] http://ngm.nationalgeographic.com/2005/11/longevity-secrets/audio-interactive

www.ingramcontent.com/pod-product-compliance
Lightning Source LLC
Chambersburg PA
CBHW040835180526
45159CB00001B/196